Valkiria Machado

Evaluation of Pharmaceutical Stability and Antimicrobial Activity

Valkiria Machado

Evaluation of Pharmaceutical Stability and Antimicrobial Activity

Semisolid topical formulations containing
essential oil of O.Gratissimum L.

ScienciaScripts

SUMMARY

Currently, microorganisms resistant to multiple antimicrobials represent a major challenge in the treatment of infections. An important strategy for reducing microbial resistance is the discovery of new substances with antibacterial and antifungal properties, mainly from natural sources. *Ocimum gratissimum,* popularly known as alfavaca and manjericão, is used in Brazil as a local antiseptic against fungi and bacteria. Due to this activity, it is one of the species considered for inclusion in the phytotherapy programme of the Unified Health System (SUS). As O. *gratissimum* causes toxicity when administered orally, the alternative to its use is in topical preparations for infected lesions, as it has been found to be active against S. *aureus, a* strain that causes skin infections. Given the population's great interest in treatments based on herbal medicines, and considering the scientifically demonstrated therapeutic potential of this plant. After the centrifugation test and preliminary stability, the semi-solid formulations (cream and cream-gel) were stored at different temperatures (ambient, refrigerator, oven and directly in sunlight) for a period of 90 days and were analysed for organoleptic characteristics, appearance, pH, viscosity and spreadability. This research has shown that it is possible to incorporate the plant's oil into formulations and that they have satisfactory physicochemical characteristics and stability, representing technological feasibility for the pharmaceutical area. The cream containing *O.gratissimum* leaf oil showed slight inhibition against *Candida Albicans* strains.

Keywords-, preliminary stability; accelerated stability; topical formulations; *candida albicans.*

SUMMARY

CHAPTER 1

INTRODUCTION

The use of plants has been widespread since the dawn of time, whether they are used in food or as therapeutic resources. Their use is based on the search for more economically accessible and less toxic alternatives (NIERO et al., 2003). Brazil is privileged with its vast wealth of plant species, which have potential in the treatment and prophylaxis of various illnesses (SIMÕES et al., 2003).

The use of medicinal plants has become a therapeutic alternative, as long as they are used with knowledge of their efficacy and safety. It should be noted that the use of medicinal plants has been increasingly accepted by the population and the medical community (OLIVEIRA, 2005; CARVALHO et al., 2008). In recent years, there has also been an increase in research and development into pharmaceutical forms containing raw materials of plant origin, thus resulting in appropriate technologies and therapies, in accordance with the prerequisites of the World Health Organisation (CALIXTO, 2005).

Herbal medicines are medicines that contain raw materials of plant origin, considered to be extraction products, such as tinctures, waxes, oils, exudates and juices. Phytotherapeutic medicines are not those that contain isolated active substances of any origin, or their combination with plant raw materials (BRASIL, 2010). In order to transform a plant raw material into a medicine, its chemical and pharmacological integrity must be preserved, thus guaranteeing its biological action and safety of use, as well as enhancing its therapeutic potential (MIGUEL & MIGUEL, 1999).

Ocimum gratissimum L. is a species of the Lamiaceae family, belonging to the *Ocimum* genus (PEREIRA & MAIA, 2007). Known as Indian basil or alfavaca (ALBUQUERQUE & ANDRADE, 1998; DI STASI et al., 2002; EHLERT, LUZ & INNECCO, 2004), it is an aromatic sub-shrub that can reach a metre in height; it originated in Asia and Africa, but its occurrence is common throughout Brazil (LORENZI & MATOS, 2000).

According to Lorenzi & Matos (2000), its leaves are used in home medicine to treat nervousness and, in infusions, as a diuretic and carminative. Its inflorescences are also used to treat digestive problems, flu, coughs, headaches, fatigue and as an expectorant (ALBUQUERQUE et al., 2007). The biological activities exerted by O. *gratissimum* are attributed to its main chemical constituents, among which are the essential oils, rich in thymol (GUENTER, 1948; VIEIRA et al, 2002), geraniol (CHARLES & SIMON, 1992; VIEIRA et al, 2002), and eugenol (BENITEZ, 2009). Also present are flavonoids such as xantomicrol and cirsimaritin (VIEIRA et al; 2002) and simple phenolic compounds (OLA et al., 2009).

Some of the biological properties of the O. *gratissimum L.* species have been scientifically proven, including: antinociceptive (RABELO et al., 2003); antibacterial (NAKAMURA et al., 1999); antagonising intestinal motility (MONTALVO & DOMÍNGUEZ, 1997) and antifungal (LEMOS et al, 2005). Current studies have demonstrated the bioactivity of O. *gratissimum* L. leaf oil against highly pathogenic organisms such as *Staphylococcus aureus, Klebisiella pneumoniae, Bacillus* spp, *Proteus mirabilis and Pseudomonas aeruginosae* (MATASYOH et al., 2007), **and of O. *gratissimum* L. inflorescence oil against *Enterococcus faecalis and Escherichia coli*** (SILVA et al., 2010).

Given that microorganisms resistant to multiple antimicrobials represent a challenge in the treatment of infections, there is a notorious need to find new substances with antimicrobial properties to be used in the fight against these microorganisms (PEREIRA, et. al., 2004). Therefore, the main objective of this study was to evaluate the pharmaceutical stability and antimicrobial activity of semi-solid topical formulations containing oil from the leaves and inflorescences of O. *gratissimum* L., and to compare the results obtained between the pharmaceutical forms.

CHAPTER 2

OBJECTIVES

2.1 GENERAL OBJECTIVE

To evaluate the pharmaceutical stability and antimicrobial activity of topical semi-solid formulations of cream containing the oil of the leaves and cream-gel containing the oil of the inflorescences of *Ocimum gratissimum* L.

2.2 SPECIFIC OBJECTIVES

- Characterise the semi-solid formulations in terms of their physical and chemical properties;
- Evaluate the stability of the emulsions (cream and cream-gel) in terms of organoleptic characteristics, pH, viscosity and spreadability;
- Compare the results of the different pharmaceutical forms developed;
- Evaluate the antifungal activity of the formulations developed against strains of *Candida sp.*

CHAPTER 3

LITERATURE REVIEW

3.1 *OCIMUM GRATISSIMUM* LINNÉ

According to taxonomy, the species O. *gratissimum* L. is classified as belonging to the Lamiaceae family, Nepetoideae subfamily, Ocimeae tribe and Ociminae subtribe (PATON et al., 2004). It is popularly known as Indian basil, alfavaca, wild alfavaca, caboclo alfavaca, Guinea alfavaca, alfavaca-da-America, alfavaca-do-campo, alfavaca-das-minas, louro, louro-de-cheiro, louro-odiroso, quioiô, quioiô-cravo and árvore-de-manjericão (ALBUQUERQUE & ANDRADE, 1998; DL STASI et al, 2002; EHLERT, LUZ & INNECCO, 2004).

Lavender is a plant that originated on the Asian continent and is used in home medicine in the form of baths, teas and is much appreciated as a condiment. The plant is an aromatic sub-shrub that grows without major problems throughout Brazil. It can reach a height of up to one metre, with oval leaves with toothed edges, varying from four to eight centimetres in length, and inflorescences with small green and purple-white flowers (JORGE et aL, 2006). It was brought to Brazil by slaves from Africa, with the aim of preserving traditional African medicine, and quickly became naturalised in the country. It is a plant that adapts to warm climates and contains a large amount of essential oils, secondary metabolites with powerful antioxidant action, acting to inhibit lipid peroxidation and neutralise free radicals (PEREIRA & MAIA, 2007).

O. *gratissimum* L. is used in Brazil as a local antiseptic against fungi and bacteria (MATOS, 1994; MORAIS et al., 2005; SILVA et al., 2006). Because it has this activity, it is one of the species considered for inclusion in the SUS phytotherapy programme (SILVA et. al., 2010). Various authors have also reported that the essential oil of O. *gratissimum* L. has analgesic and antimicrobial properties, acting on various highly pathogenic organisms (MATOS, 1998; UEDA- NAKAMURA et al., 2006; MATASYOH et al., 2007).

There are several popular uses for O. *gratissimum* L. in our country. Its flowers are used as an expectorant, digestive, calming agent and in cases of flatulence, itching and coughing (ALCÂNTARA JÚNIOR et al, 2005; ALBUQUERQUE et al, 2007). The leaves are used to treat flu (bath, decoction, syrup, infusion), mycosis (bath), bronchitis, cough (infusion, syrup), colds and as a diuretic (infusion); as a condiment (fresh), digestive, emmenagogue, expectorant, purgative and stomachic. It is also used in cases of headache (decoction, syrup), in cases of stress and tiredness (bath), flatulence, hypertension, pruritus and as a tranquilliser (DI STASI et aL, 2002; SARTORATO et aL, 2004; ALCÂNTARA JÚNIOR et aL, 2005; DUARTE et aL, 2005; FRANCO & BARROS, 2006; ALBUQUERQUE et aL, 2007; AGRA, FREITAS & BARBOSA- FILHO, 2007; LIMA et aL, 2007; OLIVEIRA & ARAÚJO, 2007).

This plant is also used in West Africa as a laxative, antiseptic, stomachic, general tonic, antidiarrhoeal, haemorrhoid, diaphoretic, ingredient in antimalarial preparations and as a treatment for coughs, fever, rheumatic pains, bronchitis and conjunctivitis (ONAJOBI, 1986; IWU, 1993). In Cuba, it is used as an antispasmodic and in cases of parasitosis, eye and ear ailments (leaves) (MONTALVO & DOMÍNGUEZ, 1997).

3.1.1 Chemical constituents

Essential oils are volatile compounds produced by plants for their survival. Secondary compounds include alkaloids, flavonoids, saponins and essential oils. Essential oils are chemical substances that perform the functions of self-defence and attracting pollinators. The plant produces essential oils in the following parts: flowers, fruit peels (called citrus fruits), leaves, small grains ("petitgrain"), roots, bark, bark resins and seeds. The "pockets" where the essential oil is encapsulated in the plant are called trichomes. These trichomes are naturally broken by the plant species, releasing the essential oil, which forms a kind of "aromatic cloud" around it (WOLFFENBÜTTEL, 2007).

Most researchers have studied the essential oil obtained from the leaves and/or aerial parts of O. *gratissimum* L. using gas chromatography coupled with mass spectrometry (GC/MS). Its composition suggests the existence of two large groups, one rich in thymol (SAINSBURY & SOFOWORA, 1971; GARCIA et aL, 1998; MARTINS et aL, 1999; YAYI et aL, 2004; TCHOUMBOUGNANG et aL, 2006) and the other rich in eugenol (JIROVETZ et aL, 2003; FREIRE, MARQUES & COSTA, 2006; TCHOUMBOUGNANG et aL, 2006). Other chemotypes have also been reported, such as ethyl cinnamate (DUBEY et aL, 2000) and geraniol (VIEIRA et aL, 2001).

Silva et al. (2007) studied the development of O. *gratissimum L. with regard to the* best harvesting time, yield and quality of its essential oils and concluded that the essential oils showed a growing increase in the majority component as the harvesting time progressed. In the leaves, the majority component is eugenol, ranging from 27.00% to 49.53% and 50.24%, and in the inflorescences the majority compound is B-selinene, ranging from 22.60% to 23.28%. CHAVES (2001) analysed the yield of essential oil from the leaves and inflorescences of lavender (O. *gratissimum* L.) subjected to increasing doses of organic fertiliser and concluded that the yield of essential oil from the leaves and inflorescences was not significant as a function of the doses of fertiliser used, but was influenced by the age of the cut and the climatic seasons for the leaves and inflorescences, with the last cut in summer showing superiority over the other climatic seasons. The general appearance of the plant and the structures of the main constituents of the essential oils and/or compounds isolated from this species can be seen in Figures 1 and 2 respectively.

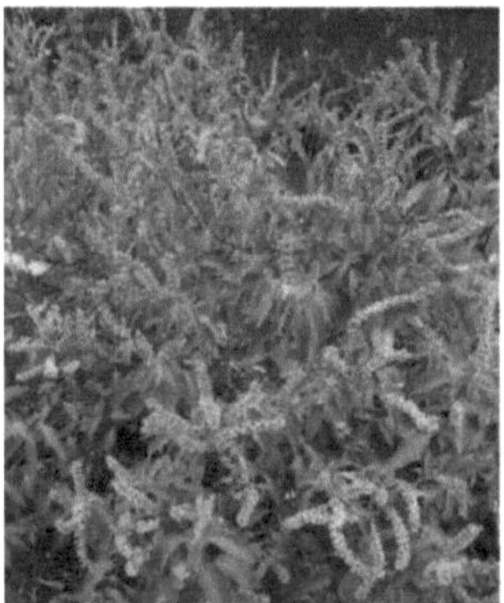

Figura 1. *Ocimum Gratissimum L.* - general appearance of the plant.

SOURCE: Silva (Personal collection)

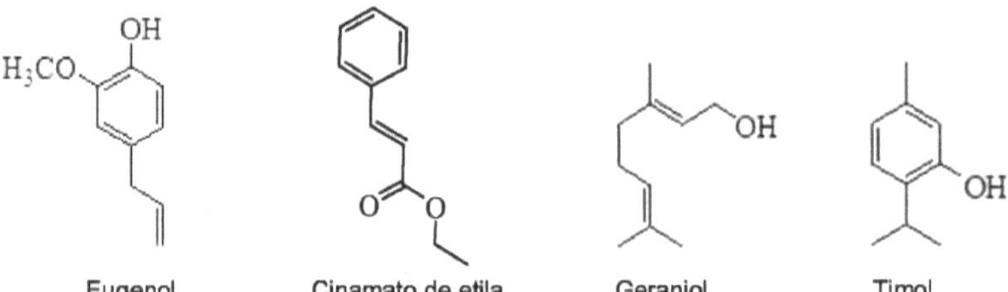

Figura 2. Major constituents of the essential oil and/or isolates of *O. gratissimum.*
(SOURCE: ADAMS, 2001; NJOKU etal., 1997; FARIA et al., 2007)

3.2 Creams and creams-gel

Creams are semi-solid pharmaceutical preparations consisting of an emulsion made up of a lipophilic phase and an aqueous phase (SILVA et al., 2006). They can be used for cosmeceutical preparations intended for external use on the skin and in products for rectal and vaginal application. They are made up of two phases closely dispersed in each other (aqueous and oily phases) in which the active ingredients are dissolved in one of the phases (GOODMAN & GILMAN, 2006).

Gel creams are emulsions made up of gel-forming polymers, which can interfere with the product's viscosity. The viscosity of an emulsion is increased depending on the

8

concentration of solids and the action of additives (PALMA & GIUDICI, 2006).

Creams and gel creams are of great clinical importance because they have medium penetration in the skin and can be used as moisturisers. In addition, creams do not retain secretions. Their active ingredients can be water-soluble and/or fat-soluble, which are able to form a homogeneous dispersion due to the addition of an emulsifying substance (GOODMAN & GILMAN, 2006).

3.3 Development of new pharmaceutical products

The most important innovation in the pharmaceutical sector takes place in product development, where there is a permanent search for increased efficacy, safety of use and reduced side effects. This process takes place by changing the characteristics of the drug to make it more effective and to cause fewer adverse or side effects; and by changing the composition of the other components of the formulation to enhance the action of the drug, such as altering the speed of its release into the body (PALMEIRA FILHO & PAN, 2003).

The initial stages of any new formulation involve studies to gather basic information on the physical and chemical characteristics of the drug to be used in a pharmaceutical form. Basic studies comprise pre-formulation work, which is necessary before starting any formulation (ALLEN JR. et aL, 2007). According to CASTILHO, MURATA & PARDI (2006), around 30% of the medicines used originate from plants, either isolated directly or produced by synthesis from a plant precursor. Natural products continue to be one of the greatest sources for discovering new drugs with antimicrobial, healing, anti-inflammatory and antineoplastic activity, among others.

In this sense, obtaining pharmaceutical forms derived from plant raw materials requires initial planning in order to properly handle the plant raw materials and other excipients in accordance with their specifications, as well as sequentially determining the technological transformation actions and monitoring the most appropriate quality control points and methodologies in accordance with current legislation and standards for the development of herbal medicines (TOLEDO et aL, 2003; OLIVEIRA et aL, 2007).

3.3.1 PHARMACEUTICAL STABILITY

Stability tests are a crucial stage in the production of pharmaceutical products, since the instability of a formulation modifies its three essential requirements: quality, safety and efficacy (KOMMANABOYINA & RHODES, 1999). The study of stability provides indications of the product's behaviour over a given period of time, in the face of the environmental conditions to which it may be subjected, from manufacture to expiry, contributing to the development of the formulation and the appropriate packaging material. In addition, stability assessment helps to improve formulations, estimate shelf life and monitor organoleptic, physical-chemical and microbiological stability, providing information on product reliability and safety (BARRY, 1983; PENA et al., 1993; BRASIL, 2004).

The product must not degrade or be irritating, and it must be compatible with the active ingredients and special additives (CARMINI & JORGE, 1989). In recent years, there has been a growing increase in the study of emulsion rheology, mainly due to its relationship with product stability (AULTON, 1988; LABA, 1993; MARTIN, 1993; SCHOTT, 1995; GALLEGOS & FRANCO, 1999; MILLER et al. 1999; LEONARDI & MAIA CAMPOS, 2001; ALMEIDA & BAHIA, 2003; LEONARDI, 2004; CORRÊA et al., 2005).

Rheological characteristics are important properties to consider when manufacturing, storing and applying topical products. Each category of product must therefore have a rheological behaviour suitable for its application, and it is advisable to know the deformation speeds of the operations it will be subjected to (LEONARDI & MAIA CAMPOS, 2001; ALMEIDA & BAHIA, 2003; CORRÊA et al., 2005). The relationship between rheology and stability is recognised as an important parameter for formulation development (TAMBURIC, 2000; CORRÊA et al., 2005).

When developing an efficient pharmaceutical form, certain parameters must be taken into account. The choice of excipients must be made through studies of the compatibility of the active ingredient with them, the bioavailability of the drug in the final formulation and its stability (KOROLKOVAS, 2002).

3.3.2 SEMI-SOLID PHARMACEUTICAL FORMS

Semisolid formulations for topical use are those intended for application to the skin. The most widely used from a pharmacotechnical point of view are gels, creams, ointments, pastes and plasters (ANSEL; POPOVICK; ALLEN, 2007).

From a physicochemical point of view, semi-solid preparations are classified as hydrogels, organogels and creams (SINKO, 2008). They can also be classified, in terms of their solubility, as single-phase lipophilic (fatty), such as hydrophobic bases, absorption bases and lipogels, or biphasic lipophilic, such as water/oil emulsions; and also as single-phase hydrophilic (miscible with water), hydrogels and biphasic hydrophilic, such as oil/water emulsions (FLORENCE & ATTWOOD, 2003). Depending on the release system, semi-solid pharmaceutical forms are further classified into dermal, transdermal occlusive patches, occlusive dressings, lipophilic materials, emulsifying bases, absorption bases, a/o emulsions, o/a emulsions, powders and humectants (AULTON, 2005).

3.4 ANTIFUNGAL ACTIVITIES

Infectious processes caused by opportunistic microbial agents are very common in Brazil, due to its geoclimatic conditions. Inextricably linked to this, there has been an increase in the emergence of bacterial and fungal infections, which occupy a prominent place in the panorama of diseases characterised as tropical (BELEM, 2002).

Resistance to antimicrobials has become a major public health problem in the contemporary world and progressive resistance has aroused worldwide concern, especially in the ongoing search for new antimicrobials (PALMEIRA et al., 2010). The *Candida* genus comprises around 150 species of fungi (SILVA et al., 2011). Candidiasis is characterised as the most common fungal infection, with C. *albicans* being its most frequent etiological agent. It is also the most prevalent species isolated from the human body, as a commensal or opportunistic pathogen (LIMA et al., 2006; SILVA et al., 2011).

Most plants have compounds that are antimicrobial and protect them from microorganisms (SILVEIRA et al., 2009). Several studies have been carried out on products of secondary plant metabolism, with the aim of finding substances with antimicrobial activity that can serve as effective therapeutic alternatives against infections by antibiotic-resistant microorganisms (ACOSTA et al., 2003).

Thus, research into extracts, fractions and essential oils from plant species is aimed at a possible rational application of active ingredients in the treatment of infections (ARAÚJO et al., 2004). Based on this, this study also set out to evaluate the antifungal potential of essential oils from the plant O. *gratissimum L.* against strains of Candida of the genus *Albicans and Glabrata* recognised as causing infectious processes.

3.5 *CANDIDA* GENERA

Yeasts of the genus *Candida* can be found in various ecosystems, such as soil, food, water and also in the normal microbiota of humans and animals (GIOLO & SVIDZINSKI, 2010). In healthy adults, *Candida sp* is found in the gastrointestinal tract in 20% to 80% of cases in men, while in women 30% are colonised in the vagina (COLOMBO & GUIMARÃES;

2003).

3.5.1 *Candida albicans*

C. albicans is the species most commonly isolated as the cause of infections, both superficial and invasive, in different anatomical sites (HAILLER, 2011). This species can be found in the oral cavity, respiratory tract, intestinal tract and vaginal cavity of humans (GOZALBO et al., 2004).

Candida albicans is a yeast that is considered a commensal in the microbiota of healthy humans. The pathogenicity of *C. albicans* is associated with the immune status of the patient in conjunction with other factors, but it can be found in more than 71 per cent of healthy individuals (NAGLIK et al., 2004).

3.5.2 *Candida glabrata*

Candida glabrata can be considered saprophytic and non-pathogenic in the normal microbiota of healthy individuals, but in the last two decades, as a consequence of immunodepressant drugs and with the advent of HIV, *C. glabrata has* increased significantly as an agent of infections in humans, becoming the second or third pathogen in cases of candidiasis, especially in hospital environments (BARCHIEESI et aL, 2005; LI, REDDING & DONGARI, 2007). Currently, *C. glabrata* is one of the most referenced species of *non-albicans Candida, as* well as having a high capacity to acquire resistance mutations to various classes of antifungal drugs (PFALLER et aL, 2012).*C. glabrata* infections are associated with patients who have been hospitalised for a long time and have previously used antimicrobial therapy (CHOW et al, 2008; SILVA et aL, 2012).

CHAPTER 4

MATERIALS AND METHODS

4.1 Reagents, Raw Materials and Equipment

The emulsions were formulated with the following raw materials: Polawax® Wax (Embacaps), Butylated hydroxytoluene (BHT) (Embacaps), Liquid Vaseline (Embacaps), Propylene glycol (Embacaps), Triethanolamine (Vetec), Preservative Solution (Phenova) (Embacaps), Silicone (Dinâmica Química Contemporânea Ltda), essential oil of *O. gratissimum* L., distilled water. The following equipment was used to assess the stability of the formulations: Brookfield rotational viscometer, model RV DVI+ with 10 speeds, MS TECNOPON potentiometer, model MPA 250, glass plates, Sterilifer oven, model SX1.1 DTMC, Cônsul refrigerator, BIOPAR water distiller, model BD5L, CHIAROTTI 2500 grater, CHIAROTTI 3 pistil, Marte precision balance, model AL 200C and centrifuge.

4.2 OBTAINING OIL FROM *OCIMUM GRATISSIMUM* L.

The essential oil from the leaves and inflorescences of *O. gratissimum* was supplied by researcher and professor Dr Lenise de Lima Silva. To obtain it, the aerial parts of *O. gratissimum* were collected on the campus of the Federal University of Santa Maria, Santa Maria - RS, between December 2006 and 2007. Witness material of this species, identified by Adelino Alvares Filho, is deposited in the herbarium of the Biology Department of UFSM under registration number 11167.

The essential oil from the leaves and inflorescences was extracted separately by hydrodistillation for 3 hours using a modified Clevenger apparatus (FARMACOPÉIA BRASILEIRA, 2010). The essential oil was stored in sealed amber glass and kept at - 4 °C until the formulations were prepared. The essential oil was analysed by gas chromatography/mass spectrometry (GC/MS).

4.3 PREPARATIONS OF SEMI-SOLID FORMULATIONS

Cream and cream-gel bases with a non-ionic character were prepared in which *O. gratissimum* oil was incorporated. The components of the cream containing *O. gratissimum* leaf oil are described in Table 1.

Table 1. Components of the non-ionic cream containing *O. gratissimum* leaf oil (COF).

PHASE	COMPONENTS	QUANTITY (%)
FO	Polawax® self-emulsifying wax	12
FO	Liquid Vaseline	3
FA	Propylene glycol	5
FA	Butylated hydroxytoluene (BHT)	0,02
FF	Preservative solution containing parabens (Phenova®)	1
FF	Triethanolamine q.s*	pH 7.0
FF	Silicone oil	5
FF	*O. gratissimum* leaf essential oil	0,2
FA	Distilled water q.s.p**	100

* Sufficient quantity of triethanolamine to obtain pH 7.0.
** Sufficient quantity to complete the volume of 100 mL.
FA= aqueous phase; FO= oily phase; FF= final phase

The carbopol dispersion was prepared by spraying the polymer onto the water using a sieve. This dispersion was left to stand for 24 hours and then mechanically stirred to obtain a homogeneous solution. The base cream was prepared using the usual technique for preparing emulsions. In a water bath, the FA components were melted in a beaker to 75°C and the FO components in a grater to 70°C. The FA was poured over the FO slowly and stirred. The preservative solution, silicone oil and O. *gratissimum oil* were incorporated into the base cream after it had cooled. After this procedure, the cream was homogenised and the pH adjusted with triethanolamine.

The components of the cream-gel containing O. *gratissimum* inflorescence oil are described in Table 2.

Table 2. Components of non-ionic cream-gel containing O. *gratissimum* inflorescence oil (CGOI).

COMPONENTS	QUANTITY (%)
6% carbopol® 940 dispersion	5
Propylene glycol	5
Butylated hydroxytoluene (BHT)	0,02
Preservative solution containing parabens (Phenova®)	1
Non-ionic base cream	7,2
Polysorbate 80 (Tween® 80)	0,8
Sorbitan monostearate (Spam® 60)	0,8
Triethanolamine q.s*	pH 7.0
Silicone oil	5
Essential oil from *O. gratissimum* inflorescences	0,2
Distilled water q.s.p**	100

* Sufficient quantity of triethanolamine to obtain pH 7.0.
** Sufficient quantity to complete the volume of 100 mL.

The base cream was prepared as follows: carbopol dispersion was added to a grater, followed by distilled water, stirring slowly. Then BHT and Spam®60, previously solubilised in Phenova®, were added. Then add the base cream, Tween® 80, propylene glycol, O.

gratissimum inflorescence oil and silicone. After this procedure, the cream-gel was homogenised and the pH adjusted with triethanolamine.

The cream-gel was prepared in triplicate, packed in double-walled plastic jars with screw caps and kept at room temperature (25 ± 2°C), in a refrigerator (5 ± 2°C), in an oven (40 ± 2°C) and exposed to sunlight (37 ± 2°C) for subsequent characterisation. The final concentration of the oil in the formulations was 0.002 mg/g of cream-gel. The components of the non-ionic base cream formulation are described in Table 3.

Table 3. Components of the non-ionic cream-gel base.

PHASE	COMPONENTS	QUANTITY (%)
FO	Polawax® self-emulsifying wax	24
FO	Cetyl alcohol	2,5
FA	Glycerine	5
FO	Decyl oleate (Cetiol® V)	6
FF	Imidazolidinyl urea 30%	2
FA	Distilled water q.s.p*	100

* Sufficient quantity to complete the volume of 100 mL. FA= aqueous phase; FO= oily phase; FF= final phase.

4.3 FORMULATION STABILITY STUDY

The stability study provides information on the product's behaviour, over a given period of time, in the face of the environmental conditions to which it may be subjected, from manufacture to expiry (ANVISA, 2004). These tests are carried out to ensure that products reach consumers in conditions suitable for use (DRAELOS, 1991).

With regard to the stability study, the semi-solid formulation was analysed for organoleptic characteristics, appearance, pH, viscosity and spreadability.

4.3.1. Organoleptic characteristics

The analysis of organoleptic characteristics is a procedure used to evaluate the product and provide parameters to analyse the state of the sample under study in order to verify alterations such as changes in colour, odour, phase separation and precipitation (ANVISA, 2008). The physical characteristics, i.e. appearance, colour and odour, of the samples stored in an oven (ES), refrigerator (GE) and directly in sunlight (LS) were visually analysed and compared with the samples stored at room temperature (T.A), which were used as a standard.

Table 4 - Scale used to assess organoleptic characteristics.

SCALE	ASPECT
1	Normal, satisfactory condition (no change in colour or appearance)

2	Slight change in some aspect of the sample's appearance, colour and odour
3	Incorporation of air, start of development of colour or odour,
4	Beginning of phase separation of the sample, noticeable colouration, product with altered odour
5	Separated phases, strongly coloured product and/or with an unpleasant odour

The organoleptic characteristics and homogeneity of the formulations were observed for 90 days. It should be noted that the initial assessment will be carried out after 24 hours of preparation, together with the Centrifugation Test.

4.3.2 Determining pH

Large variations in pH indicate a possible instability of the formulation, considering that it is a chemical parameter and can indicate a lack of stability between the ingredients of the formulations, compromising the efficacy and safety of the product (BRASIL, 2004). To determine the pH of the formulations, a potentiometer calibrated with a pH 4.0 and 7.0 buffer solution was used. The readings were taken through direct contact of the electrode with the samples (ALVES, 2006). The results were expressed as the average of the three determinations. The readings were taken at T. A.

4.3.3 Determining viscosity

Viscosity is the product's resistance to deformation or flow, which depends on the physical-chemical characteristics and temperature conditions of the material. It can be determined using a rotary viscometer, which consists of measuring the amount required to rotate a spindle immersed in a fluid (BRASIL, 2008). Evaluating this parameter helps determine whether a product has the appropriate consistency or fluidity and can indicate whether stability is adequate, i.e. it provides an indication of the product's behaviour over time (ANVISA, 2004).

The rheological characteristics of the semi-solid formulations were assessed using a Brookfield rotational viscometer, model RV DVI+ with 10 speeds (100 rpm speed using spindle 29). The rheograms were constructed by graphing the shear rate as a function of shear stress. Rheological behaviour was also monitored according to the relationship between viscosity and shear rate (ALVES, 2006).

4.3.4 Spreadability

In semi-solid pharmaceutical forms, this parameter is important for monitoring changes in the formulation's ability to spread or cover a certain area, which can make it easier or more difficult to apply (BUGNOTTO et al., 2006). To determine spreadability, the parallel plate method proposed by De Paula et al., 1988, will be used.

A circular glass mould-plate (diameter = 20 cm; thickness = 0.2 cm), with a central hole 1.2 cm in diameter, was placed on a glass support-plate (20 cm x 20 cm). A sheet of graph paper was placed underneath. The sample was inserted into the hole in the plate and the surface levelled with a spatula. The mould-plate was then carefully removed. A glass plate of a predetermined weight was placed on top of the sample. After one minute, the surface area covered was calculated by measuring the diameter in two opposite positions and then calculating the average diameter. This procedure was repeated, adding new plates at one-minute intervals and recording the surface area covered after each determination. The spreadability (Ei), determined at 25°C, was calculated using the equation below:

$Ei = (d^2.\pi)/4,$ where:

Ei = spreadability of the sample for weight i (mm)$;^2$

D = average diameter (mm);

The spreadability values as a function of the weights added were determined by taking three measurements and calculating the average between them. The analyses were carried out in triplicate. It should be noted that the values used to draw up the graphs and tables refer to the weight of the plates (147.026g) in which all the samples were read.

4.3. 5Centrifugation test

Centrifugation increases particle mobility and anticipates possible signs of instability, such as precipitation, phase separation, compact sediment formation and coalescence (BRASIL, 2005). Centrifugation produces stress in the sample, simulating an increase in the force of gravity, increasing the mobility of the particles and anticipating possible instabilities. These can be observed in the form of precipitation, phase separation, compact sediment formation and coalescence, among others (PROENÇA et al, 2006).

Five grams (5 g) of each sample were added to a specific centrifuge test tube, weighed on a semi-analytical balance and centrifuged for 30 minutes at a speed of 3,000 rpm with three readings for each sample, as recommended in ANVISA's Stability Guide (2004).The occurrence of instability indicates the need for reformulation. The formulations that were stable in this test were submitted to the Preliminary Stability Test (ISAAC et aL, 2008).

4.3. 6Preliminary stability test   (freeze-thaw cycle)

The aim of preliminary stability testing is to help and guide the choice of formulations. Thus, it is necessary to use extreme temperature conditions to accelerate possible reactions between the components of the formulation and the appearance of signs that need to be observed and analysed according to the specific characteristics of each product (BRASIL, 2004). The freezing and thawing cycle was carried out in accordance with the ANVISA Stability Guide (2004). The samples were subjected to a two-week cycle at alternating temperatures, at regular intervals of time, every twenty-four hours, at a temperature of 40°C in an electric oven, and at a temperature of 5°C in a refrigerator. Readings were taken before the start of the test and at the end of the cycle (15 days).

4.3.7 Accelerated stability test

It is a study designed to accelerate the chemical degradation or physical changes of a pharmaceutical product through the use of forced storage conditions (BRASIL, 2004). The samples considered stable by the preliminary test were subjected to variable temperature conditions, i.e. they were heated in an electric oven (40 ± 2°C), cooled in a refrigerator (5 ± 2°C), at room temperature (25 ± 2°C) and in direct sunlight for 90 days. Sample readings were taken before the start of the test (24 hours after the formulations were prepared), on the 30th, 60th and 90th days.

4.5 SUSCEPTIBILITY TESTS

4.5.1 Microorganisms

The clinical isolate has been identified by molecular techniques and the cultures of the isolates have been replicated on Sabouraud dextrose agar plus Chloramphenicol.

4.4.2 Agar diffusion disc

The antifungal activity of the pure oil in the cream and cream-gel pharmaceutical forms was assessed using the disc diffusion technique according to CLSI protocol M44-A2 (2008). The strains were grown on Sabouraud dextrose agar for 24 hours at 37°C in a bacteriological incubator. The inoculum is a dilution of 5 colonies of the microorganism in sterile 0.85%

saline solution and compared to the McFarland scale of 0.5 ($1\text{-}5\text{x}10^6$ cells/mL). The Mueller Hinton agar medium used in the test was supplemented with 2% glucose for better fungal development and 0.5 pg/ml methylene blue, resulting in a pH of 7.2- 7.4. After standardising the inoculum, it was sown on the surface of the agar using a sterile *swab* in three different directions. Next, 6 mm diameter filter paper discs, with a distance of 24 mm between discs, were inserted into the agar surface and then 10 pL of the pure oil and the formulations were inoculated. The control was carried out using impregnated discs

with nystatin cream. The plates were inverted and incubated for 20-24 hours at 35°C. The result was obtained by measuring the halo of inhibition formed around the disc (CLINICAL AND LABORATORY STANDARDS INSTITUTE, 2008).

4.5 STATISTICAL ANALYSES OF THE RESULTS

The statistical methodology of the data includes descriptive analysis of variables such as the mean, standard deviation, coefficient of variation, correlation studies, simple linear regression and Tukey's test, considering significance levels of <0.05.

CHAPTER 5

RESULTS

5.1 Preliminary stability

After 24 hours of preparing the formulations, the pH remained at 7.52 ± 0.01 and 7.62 ± 0.00 for the cream containing leaf oil (COF) and the cream-gel containing inflorescence oil (CGOI), respectively (Table 7). Figure 2 shows that the COF initially had a white colour, while the CGOI had a slightly yellow colour, both with a shiny, homogeneous appearance. All the formulations had a characteristic odour of the *O. gratissimum* plant.

In the macroscopic analysis of the formulations, the appearance, colour and odour of the samples remained unchanged, except for the CGOI formulation, which had a slight colour change compared to its initial colour (Figure 3). The viscosity readings for the formulations were taken at a speed of 100 rpm using spindle 29. The initial viscosity values found for COF and CGOI were 1656 ± 228 and 2666 ± 85 mPa.s, respectively (Table 8). As for spreadability, the initial test results obtained were 2055 ± 46 and 3002 ± 148 for COF and CGOI, respectively (Table 9).

The formulations under study did not show any phase separation in the centrifugation test carried out 24 hours after preparation. They were all considered stable and were therefore subjected to the freeze-thaw cycle, characterising preliminary stability. The formulations developed proved to be stable in the preliminary stability tests. No changes in colour, odour or phase separation parameters were observed for COF. For CGOI, the freeze-thaw cycle led to the appearance of a yellowish colour at the end of the 15 days (Figure 3).

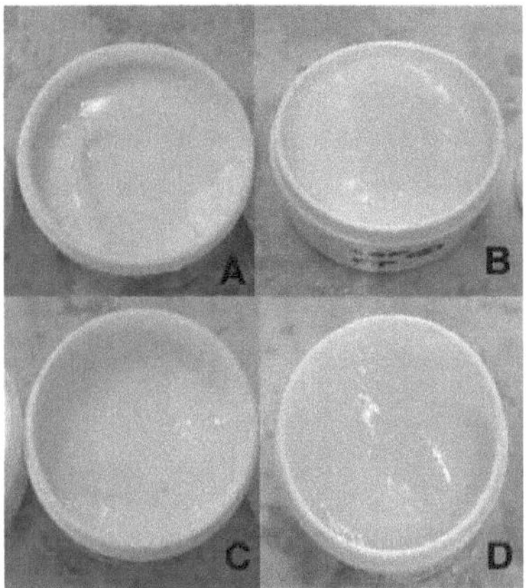

Figure 3 - COF 24 hours after preparation (A), COF 15 days after freeze-thaw cycle (B), CGOI 24 hours after preparation (C), CGOI 15 days after freeze-thaw cycle (D).

The pH values obtained for the formulations submitted to the preliminary test were 6.37 ± 0.00 and 7.65 ± 0.00 for COF and CGOI, respectively, at the end of 15 days (Table 7). It is worth noting that the COF formulation significantly reduced the pH ($p<0.001$), which did not occur with the CGOI formulation after 15 days, when compared to the result obtained after 24 hours of preparation. The viscosity results observed for COF and CGOI were 5323 ± 112 and 5266 ± 23 mPa.s, corresponding to an increase in relation to the initial value (Table 8). With regard to spreadability, 2821 ± 1132 and 3089 ± 351 were the results obtained for COF and CGOI after 15 days, which is not statistically different from the initial values (Table 9).At the end of the freeze-thaw cycle, the CGOI formulation proved to be more stable with regard to pH values. Both formulations did not undergo significant changes in spreadability values after 15 days, while viscosity values changed significantly.

5.2 Accelerated stability

Once the preliminary stability study had been completed, the samples were subjected to the accelerated stability test. The formulations stored at room temperature (T.A), in an oven (ES), in sunlight (LS) and in a refrigerator (GE) were analysed for pH, organoleptic characteristics, viscosity and spreadability after 30, 60 and 90 days of the experiment. In terms of organoleptic characteristics, the COF formulation showed a slight change in colour from the formulations stored in the L.S. at 60 days. This formulation also had a slight change in odour at 90 days. It is worth noting that the formulation stored in ES, T.A and GE showed some instability in the formulation after 60 days, as phase separation began to be observed in different proportions according to the condition to which it was exposed. The CGOI formulation showed colour changes in the formulations stored in L.S and ES from 60 days onwards. The formulations intensified their yellow colour and showed a slight change in odour, which continued until 90 days. The samples stored in T.A. showed a change in colour only at the end of 90 days. The CGOI formulation exposed to GE showed no odour and no colour change, but showed slight destabilisation in its formula at the end of the 60-day test (Figure 4).

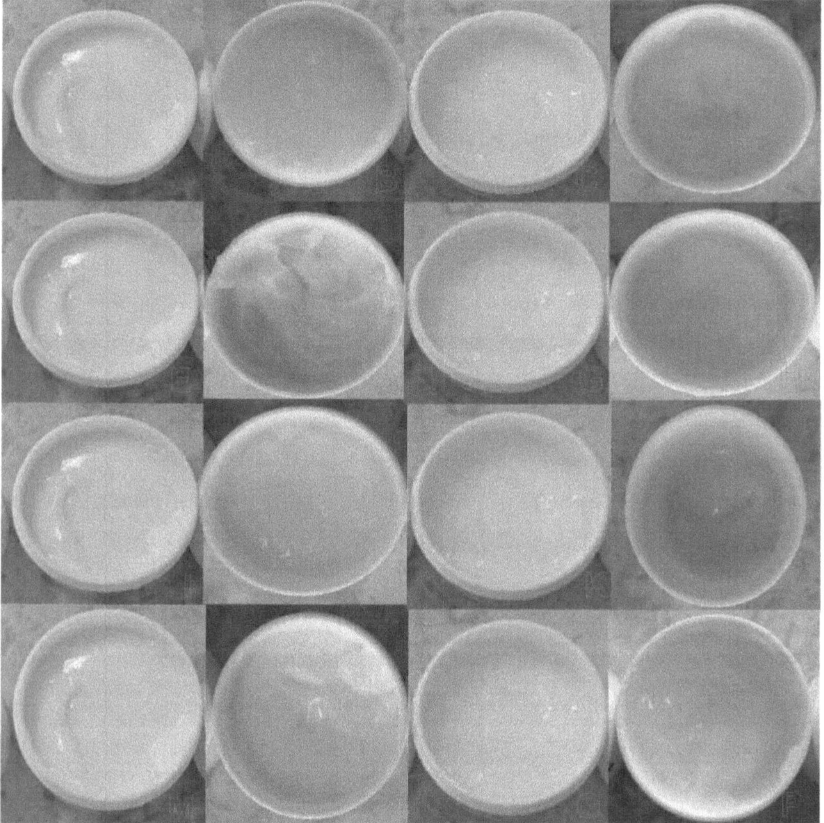

Figure 4 - COF 24 hours after preparation (A, E, I, M), COF 90 days after storage in T.A (B), COF 90 days after exposure to L.S (F), COF 90 days after storage in ES (J), COF 90 days after storage in GE (N), CGOI 24 hours after preparation (C, G, K, O), CGOI 90 days after storage in T. A (D), CGOI 90 days after storage in ES (L), CGOI 90 days after storage in GE (P).A (D), CGOI 90 days after exposure to L.S (H), CGOI 90 days after storage in ES (L), CGOI 90 days after storage in GE (P).

	ORGANOLEPTIC CHARACTERISTICS	
TIME	COF	CGOI
24 hours	1	1

15 day defrost cycle	1	2
30 days T.A	1	1
30 days L.S	1	1
30 days ES	1	1
30 days GE	1	1
60 days T.A	2	1
60 days L.S	2	2
60 days ES	2	2
60 days GE	2	2
90 days T.A	2	2
90 days L.S	2	2
90 days ES	2	2
90 days GE	2	2

1 Normal, satisfactory condition (no change in colour or appearance).
2 A slight change in some aspect of the sample's appearance, colour and odour.

Table 6- Organoleptic characteristics of the formulations during the preliminary and accelerated stability tests.

The pH values of the COF samples stored in all the conditions tested (T.A, L.S, GE and ES) fell at 30, 60 and 90 days when compared to the initial values. In the CGOI samples stored in L.S and GE, the pH values fluctuated, as they increased significantly ($p<0.001$) at 30 days, decreased at 60 days and increased again significantly ($p<0.001$) at 90 days compared to the initial values.

The CGOI samples stored in ES also showed significant changes ($p<0.001$), fluctuating their values, which increased from 30 days onwards and reduced their pH at 60 and 90 days of the experiment compared to the initial values. The CGOI samples stored in T.A. increased significantly at all analysis times.

	pH ± SD	
TIME / CONDITIONS TESTED	**COF**	**CGOI**
24 hours	7,52 ± 0,01	7,62 ± 0,00
15 days	6,37 ± 0,00*	7,65 ± 0,00
30 days T.A	6,47 ±0,01*	7,73 ±0,01*
30 days L.S	6,33 ± 0,00*	7,72 ±0,01*
30 days ES	5,68 ±0,01*	7,72 ± 0,02*
30 days GE	7,15 ±0,00*	7,87 ± 0,00*
60 days T.A	6,63 ±0,01*	7,81 ± 0,00*
60 days L.S	5,71 ±0,01*	7,40 ± 0,00*
60 days ES	4,82 ± 0,00*	7,48 ± 0,00*
60 days GE	6,72 ± 0,00*	7,55 ± 0,00*
90 days T.A	6,13 ±0,01*	7,66 ± 0,00*
90 days L.S	6,21 ± 0,00*	7,69 ±0,01*
90 days ES	5,62 ±0,01*	7,51 ± 0,03*
90 days GE	6,89 ±0,01*	7,63 ±0,01*

Table 7. pH values obtained for the COF and CGOI formulations during the preliminary and

accelerated stability tests.

* Statistically significant values (p<0.05) when compared to their initial results.

Table 8. Viscosity values (mPa.s) obtained for COF and CGOI during the

TIME / CONDITIONS TESTED	VISCOSITY (mPa.s) ± SD	
	COF	CGOI
24 hours	1656 ±228	2666 ± 85
15 days	5323±112*	5266 ± 23*
30 days T.A	5673±109*	5480±17*
30 days L.S	5416 ±5*	5243±11*
30 days ES	2130±104*	5246 ±51*
30 days GE	3990 ± 270*	6063 ± 23*
60 days T.A	5133±188*	5600 ± 0*
60 days L.S	5506±177*	1886 ±40*
60 days ES	2290±108*	4106 ±70*
60 days GE	4380 ± 545*	5540±103*
90 days T.A	4096 ± 95*	3670±117*
90 days L.S	4323 ± 57*	2256±150*
90 days ES	2233 ± 57*	2650±132
90 days GE	2600 ± 200	3296 ± 5*

preliminary and accelerated stability tests.

* Statistically significant values (p<0.05) when compared to their initial results.

Comparing the initial results with the final viscosity results, it was found that the COF and CGOI formulations generally increased their viscosity values under all the conditions analysed. Exceptions to this pattern were observed with COF at 90 days stored in GE and CGOI at 90 days stored in ES, where no changes in viscosity were detected in relation to their initial values. In addition, there was a significant reduction in the viscosity of CGOI formulations exposed to L.S from 60 days onwards.

Table 9. Spreadability values obtained for COF and CGOI during the preliminary and accelerated stability tests.

TIME / CONDITIONS TESTED	SPREADABILITY ± DP	
	COF	CGOI
24 hours	2055 ± 46	3002 ±148
15 days	2821 ±1132	3089 ± 351
30 days T.A	3125 ±425*	2041 ± 0*
30 days L.S	2907 ± 583	2171 ±505
30 days ES	2700 ± 695	1731 ±311
30 days GE	3429 ± 443*	2598 ±231*
60 days T.A	1810±134	1635 ±303
60 days L.S	3022 ± 300*	2831 ± 597
60 days ES	2659±1091	2096 ± 780
60 days GE	3189 ±393*	2610 ±69*
90 days T.A	1701 ±204	2296 ±317*

90 days L.S	2003±138	2833 ± 357
90 days ES	3600 ± 379	2467 ± 286
90 days GE	2418±114	2346±108*

* Statistically significant values (p<0.05) when compared to their initial results.

Both samples stored in T.A. showed significant changes (p<0.05) in spreadability after 30 days. These changes were not maintained at 60 days for both samples. However, reductions were seen again for CGOI at 90 days in this condition.

The COF samples exposed to L.S showed an increase in spreadability only after 60 days, which was not observed in the other test periods. The CGOI sample exposed to L.S and ES did not change significantly throughout the tests. No changes were observed in the spreadability of COF exposed to ES.

The COF samples stored in GE increased in spreadability over 30 and 60 days when compared to the initial results. The CGOI sample in the same condition showed a reduction in spreadability at all observation times.

5.1 SUSCEPTIBILITY TESTS

The COF and CGOI formulations were tested against strains of *C. albicans* and a clinical isolate of *C. glabrata*. The results of the inhibition halo found for the gel cream containing essential oil from *Ocimum gratissumum* influorescences against the C. *albicans* species are described in Table 10.

Table 10 - Inhibition halo against *Candida albicans* ATCC14053.

CGOI SAMPLES	INHIBITION HALO ± SD
Cream-gel with inflorescence oil with preservative	5,33 ± 3,26
Cream-gel with preservative-free inflorescence oil	0±0
Preservative-free cream-gel base	0±0

Table 11 - Inhibition halo against the clinical isolate of *C.glabrata.*

CGOI SAMPLES	INHIBITION HALO ± SD
Cream and oil from inflorescences with preservative	0±0
Cream-gel with preservative-free inflorescence oil	0±0
Preservative-free cream-gel base	0±0

Table 12 - Inhibition halo against *Candida albicans* ATCC14053.

COF SAMPLES	INHIBITION HALO ± SD

Cream with preservative-free leaf oil	0±0
Cream with preservative-free leaf oil	0±0
Preservative-free base cream	0±0

Table 13 - Inhibition halo against a clinical isolate of *C.glabrata.*

COF SAMPLES	INHIBITION HALO ± SD
Cream with preservative-free leaf oil	0±0
Cream-gel with preservative-free leaf oil	0±0
Preservative-free cream-gel base	0±0

The CGOI formulation without preservative did not inhibit the growth of the *C.albicans* strains, *and the* same can be seen with the cream gel base formulation with the preservative, which also did not show an inhibition halo (Figure 5).

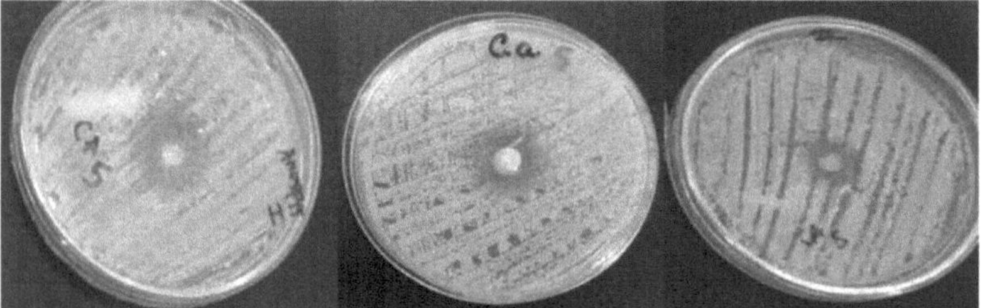

Figure 5 - Inhibition halo of the cream-gel containing *Ocimum gratissimum* oil against *Candida Albicans* ATCC 14053 strains.

CHAPTER 6

DISCUSSION

The stability of creams and lotions, i.e. emulsions, is defined as the period in which the product maintains, within the specified limits and within the period of storage and use (the latter being the product's expiry date) the stability of the product.
properties and characteristics that it possessed when it was manipulated (LEONARDI & CAMPOS, 2001). It is not easy to find quick and sensitive methods to determine the stability of an emulsion. When stored on shelves under normal storage conditions, it usually takes prolonged periods before progressive signs appear that can determine the instability of the cream. It is therefore necessary to accelerate instability by subjecting the cream to stress conditions (RIEGER, 2001).

Emulsions represent cosmetic and/or pharmaceutical vehicles that are widely used, as they allow for the incorporation of a wide range of active ingredients, both water-soluble and fat-soluble, as well as generally showing good acceptance when their sensory characteristics are taken into account during formulation design (OTTO et al., 2009). There are several factors that can compromise the physicochemical and microbiological stability of an emulsified system, such as: choice of incompatible constituents, type and concentration of emulsifiers, stirring speed, heating and cooling time, phase quantities, storage temperature and environment and contamination by microorganisms (IDSON, 1993; RIEGER, 1996; SCHUELLER & RORMANOWSKI, 2000; ALVAREZ et al, 2007).

It is well known that sensory evaluation is an extremely important tool for guaranteeing a product's sales success. Nowadays, a technical professional shouldn't just think about the stability of the final product, as it's very important to think about the well-being that the application of the product will offer the consumer. The sensory characteristics people want can be achieved with the right combination of liquid emollients and waxes in the product formulation (LUKIC et al., 2012). These components have a major influence on the sensory characteristics and the acceptability or perceived benefits of the cosmetic product by consumers (PARENTE et al., 2010).

Centrifugation can be used to observe the separation of the internal phase. When applied carefully, centrifugation is a useful tool for assessing the stability of emulsions (RIEGER, 2001). After the freeze-thaw cycle, the COF samples remained stable, with no change in colour, odour or phase separation parameters, and there was a significant reduction in pH values after 15 days. pH control is essential because it prevents undesirable skin reactions to the product, such as irritation, redness, itching and others (LEONARDI, GASPAR and CAMPOS, 2002). Determining the viscosity of emulsions is a suitable criterion for estimating their quality, but it is not carried out using absolute viscosity values, but rather changes in viscosity during storage (RIEGER, 2001). COF showed no significant difference in viscosity at the end of the freeze-thaw cycle. These results are in line with those obtained by Lima et al. (2008), where O/W emulsions containing babassu oil showed stability in the thermal stress test.

The CGOI samples were also stable in the freeze-thaw cycle, as there was no phase separation or change in the odour of the formulations, but the colour changed from white to slightly yellowish, which could make it unacceptable to consumers. In terms of viscosity, the CGOI showed a significant increase at the end of the 15 days of preliminary tests. With regard to the spreadability of the formulations in the freeze-thaw cycle, both kept their spreadability values stable. Ferrari (2002) states that when carrying out preliminary stability tests, the results cannot be analysed in isolation. Therefore, considering that the pH, viscosity and spreadability values of the samples remained within acceptable standards, the samples were submitted to the accelerated stability test.

The pH corresponds to the hydrogen concentration of the skin's surface and is an important functional indicator of the skin. This is why the skin has a slightly acidic pH (4.6 - 5.8), which contributes to protection against bacteria and fungi on its surface. In addition, skin secretions have an appreciable buffering capacity, which is an important property since the pH of the skin is often altered as a result of the use of inappropriate topical products, which can expose the skin to a series of aggressive agents, especially microorganisms. Determining and controlling the pH of the formulations developed is extremely useful, not least to avoid the use of unsuitable topical products, since skin contact with formulations containing aggressive substances - such as detergents - is frequent.

In the COF and CGOI formulations, it was possible to see that the pH values changed significantly after 90 days in all the conditions tested. This result is in line with the study by Pianovski et al. (2008), in which cosmetic emulsions prepared with Pequi oil (*Ca/yocar brasiliense)* showed significant differences in pH value during the 90 days at different times and temperatures.

Rheological analyses as a function of temperature are fundamental for obtaining information on the physical stability of the product, as well as its consistency. Emulsion rheology is a direct manifestation of the interaction of forces occurring in the system. Creaming, sedimentation, coalescence and flocculation are processes that occur in emulsions and can be investigated through rheology (MOSTEFA *et al,* 2006; TADROS, 1999; 2004).

In the present study, the formulation with the lowest viscosity was the COF stored in the oven, the formation of lumps was noticeable and the volume of the creams decreased. Water evaporation probably occurred at high temperatures, triggering the process of evaporation of the water contained in the formulations, increasing their consistency index.

CGOI's viscosity values increased significantly when stored at T.A. and GE after 90 days. The viscosity values decreased significantly when stored in L.S and ES. The COF formulation suffered a significant increase in all the conditions tested. It can therefore be inferred that high temperatures influence the decrease in viscosity of the aforementioned formulation. As for the COF formulations, there was no influence on their stability at the different temperatures tested. Both the COF and CGOI formulations differed statistically when stored in ES.

All the formulations tested maintained good spreadability during the 90-day experiment, which is one of the essential characteristics of pharmaceutical forms intended for topical application. Spreadability is closely related to the application of these formulations at the site of action and is characterised by the fluidity of the formulation obtained, making it possible to choose the most suitable one and assess its performance and consumer acceptance (MARTINS, CORTEZ & FELIPE, 2008).

Among the formulations tested, COF stored in ES was the formulation with the highest spreadability at the end of the study. The formulation with the lowest spreadability at 90 days was COF stored in T.A.

Comparing the samples stored in ES with those stored in T.A., it was observed that the COF samples obtained higher spreadability results in ES. It can therefore be inferred that high temperatures influence the spreadability of the COF formulation. These results corroborate the data obtained by Pereira and Frasson (2007), where the highest spreadability value was found for samples of anionic cream containing glycolic extract of *Aloe Vera* stored in ES.

According to Somasundaran et al. (2007), ionic silicones can be used as rheological property modifiers, helping to increase viscosity. In this study, silicone was also added to the formulation, which improved the rheological properties of viscosity and spreadability.

With regard to antimicrobial activity, the cream-gel with the essential oil from the inflorescences of *Ocimum gratissimum L.* did not show antifungal activity against the clinical isolate of *C. glabrata,* but showed slight inhibition against the *C. albicans strain* at the formulation concentration tested.

Therefore, although the results obtained are not considered promising, the reports of the antimicrobial properties of species of the genus *Ocimum,* together with the advantages of using drugs from natural sources, justify the importance of continuing studies into the antimicrobial activity of the essential oil of *Ocimum gratissimum* against other microorganisms. Considering that a promising resource for the discovery of new antifungal agents with fewer side effects comes from plants used in folk medicine to treat fungal infections, the oils obtained from which have served as the basis for various therapeutic applications.

Further studies are needed to better verify and determine antimicrobial activity, stability against different packaging and dosage of active ingredients, in order to obtain more detailed information on the shelf life of products containing O. *gratissimum* oil and extract.

CHAPTER 7

CONCLUSION

Based on the results obtained in this study, it was concluded that incorporating O. *gratissimum L.* oil into semi-solid bases is feasible. However, the addition of the oil increases the rheological characteristics of the formulations. With regard to organoleptic aspects, it was possible to notice slight changes in the odour and colour of the formulations, suggesting the need for prior treatments, such as increasing the concentration or even changing the antioxidant agent to stabilise the natural constituents. Comparing the two formulations, it was found that CGOI showed better stability than COF at the end of the freeze-thaw cycle. This shows that sudden temperature variations do not influence the stability of this formulation. COF showed better stability over the 90 days of the experiment under the different conditions tested, in terms of spreadability and viscosity when compared to CGOI. In terms of tested stability, the cream containing O. *gratissimum* leaf oil proved to be more stable in the tests than the gel cream containing oil from the inflorescences.

In terms of antimicrobial activity, the essential oil from the inflorescences of O. *gratissimum L.* proved to potentiate the action of the preservative in the cream-gel formulation. Therefore, further studies are of fundamental importance in order to understand its action against other micro-organisms.

CHAPTER 8

BIBLIOGRAPHICAL REFERENCES

ACOSTA, M.; GONZÁLEZ, M.; ARAQUE, M.; VELAZCO, E.; KHOURL. N.; ROJAS, L.; USUBILLAGA, A. 2003. Composición química de los aceites esenciales de *Ocimum basilicum L. var basilicum, O. basilicum L.* var purpurenscens, *O. gratissimum L., y O. tenuiflorum L.,* y su efecto antimicrobiano sobre bactérias multirresistentes de origen nosocomial. **Revista Facultad de Farmacia,** 45: 19-24.

ADAMS, R. P. **Identification of essential oil components by gas chromatography/quadrupole mass spectroscopy.** Illinois: Allured, 2001.

NATIONAL HEALTH SURVEILLANCE AGENCY. **Stability guide for cosmetic products.** Brasília: ANVISA, 2004. 52p. (Thematic Series, v.1). Available at: http://www.anvisa.gov.br/divulga/public/series/cosmeticos.pdf. Accessed on: 14 September 2014.

AGRA, M. F.; FREITAS, P. F.; BARBOSA-FILHO, J. M. Synopsis of plants known as medicinal and poisonous in the Northeast of Brazil. **Revista Brasileira de Farmacognosia,** v. 17, p. 114-140, 2007.

ALBUQUERQUE, U. P. et al. Medicinal plants of the caatinga (semi-arid) vegetation of NE Brazil: A quantitative approach. **Journal of Ethnopharmacology,** v. 114, p. 325-354, 2007.

ALBUQUERQUE, U. P.; ANDRADE, L. H. C. El género *Ocimum* L. (Lamiaceae) en el Nordeste del Brasil. **Anales Jardín Botánico de Madrid,** v. 56, n. 1, p.43-64, 1998.

ALCÂNTARA JÚNIOR, J. P. et al. Ethnobotanical and ethnopharmacological survey of medicinal plants in the municipality of Itaberaba-BA for cultivation and preservation. **Sitientibus Série Ciências Biológicas, v.** 5, n. 1, p. 39-44, 2005.

ALLEN JR, L. V.; POPOVICH, N. G.; ANSEL, H.C. **Pharmaceutical Forms and Drug Delivery Systems.** 8th ed. Porto Alegre: Editora Artmed, 2007.

ALMEIDA, I.F, BAHIA, M.F. Rheology: interest and applications in the cosmetic-pharmaceutical area. **Cosmetics & Toiletries.** 2003; 15(3):96-100.

ALVES, M. P. **Development and stability assessment of dermatological bases. Influence of absorption promoters on the transdermal permeation of piroxicam.** Master's dissertation. Postgraduate Programme in Pharmaceutical Sciences and Technology: Federal University of Santa Maria-UFSM, 1996.

. **Plastic pharmaceutical forms containing nimesulide nanocapsules, nanospheres and nanoemulsions: development, characterisation and evaluation of *in vitro* skin permeation.** Thesis (Doctorate). Postgraduate Programme in Pharmaceutical Sciences: Faculty of Pharmacy, Federal University of Rio Grande do Sul - UFRGS, Porto Alegre-RS, 2006.

ANSEL H. C.; POPOVICH N. G.; ALLEN L. V. JR. **Pharmaceutical forms and drug delivery systems.** 8 ed. Porto Alegre: Artmed, 2007.

ARAÚJO, J. C. L. V.; LIMA, E. O.; CEBALLOS, B. S. O.; FREIRE, K. R. L.; SOUZA, E. L.; FILHO. L. S. Antimicrobial action of essential oils on microorganisms potentially causing opportunistic infections. **Revista de patologia tropical,** Vol. 33 (1), 55-64, Jan-Jun, 2004.

ASBILL, C. S.; MICHNIAK, B. B. Percutaneous penetration enhancers: local versus transdermal activity. **Pharmaceutical Science & Technology Today,** v.3, n.1, p.36- 41, 2000.

AULTON M. E. **Delineamento de formas farmacêuticas.** 2. ed. Porto Alegre: Artmed, 677p, 2005.

. Pharmaceutics: The Science of dosage form design. New York: **Churchill Livingstone;** 1988. p.57-73.

BARCHIEESI F, SPREGNINI E, TOMASSETTI S, ARZENI D, GINNINI D, SCALISE G. Comparison of the fungicidal activities of caspofungin and amphotericin B against *Candida glagrata.* **Antimicrobial Agents and Chemotherapy** 2005; 49(12) 49894992.

BARREIRO, E. J.; BOLZANI, V.S. Biodiversity: a potential source for drug discovery. **Química Nova,** v. 32, n. 3, p. 679-688, 2009.

BARRY B.W. Dermatological formulations: percutaneous absorption. New York: **Mareei Dekker;** 1983. p.351-403.

BRAZIL. **Technical Report No.º 01, of 15 July 2008** - Clarification on item 2.9 of the annex to Resolution RE No. 1 of 29/07/2005, which deals with the Guide for carrying out stability studies Agência Nacional de Vigilância Sanitária. Executive Power, Brasília, DF. Federal Official Gazette, 15 July 2008.

. Ministry of Health. National Health Surveillance Agency. **Stability guide for cosmetic products.** Brasília, DF: ANVISA; 2004. 52p.

. Ministry of Health. National Health Surveillance Agency. **Stability guide for cosmetic products.** Brasília, 45p, 2004.

. Ministry of Health. National Health Surveillance Agency. Collegiate Board Resolution No. 14 of 31 March 2010. Provides for the registration of herbal medicines. OFFICIAL GAZETTE, 05. April, 2010.

. **Resolution no. 01 of 29 July 2005.** Guide to conducting stability studies. [Internet]. National Health Surveillance Agency. Poder Executivo, Brasília, DF, Diário Oficial da União, 01 August, 2005.

BENITEZ, N. P.; MELÉNDEZ LEÓN, E. M.; STASHENKO, E. E. Eugenol and methyl eugenol chemotypes of essential oil of species *ocimum gratissimum L.* and *Ocimum campechianum* Mill. from Colombia. **Jounal of Chromatographic Science, v.** 47, n. 9, p. 800-803, oct. 2009.

BELEM, L .F. **Epidemiological study of pityriasis versicolor in the state of Paraíba and chemical and antifungal evaluation of natural and synthetic products against its etiological agent.** João Pessoa, 178 p. [PhD thesis - Postgraduate programme in bioactive natural and synthetic products - Pharmaceutical Technology Laboratory - UFPB], 2002.

BUGNOTTO, C. SOARES, G. LAPORTA, L. V.; ALVES, M. P.; SCHMIDT, C. A.; LIMBERGER, J. B. Stability Study of Topical Formulations Containing Propolis. **Disc Scientia.** Series: Health Sciences, Santa Maria, v. 7, n. 1, p. 1-12, 2006.

CALIXTO, J. B. Twenty-five Years of Research on Medicinal plants in Latin America: A personal view. **Journal of Ethnopharmacology,** v. 100, n. 1-2, p. 131-134, 2005.

CARMINI, M. O.; JORGE, M. C. G. Cosmetic creams and emulsions: basic concepts. **Cosmetics & Toiletries,** São Paulo, v. 1, n. 5. p. 13 - 22, Sep/Oct, 1989.

CARVALHO, A. C. B.; BALBINO, E. E.; MACIEL, A.; PERFEITO, J. P. S. Status of the registration of herbal medicines in Brazil. **Brazilian Journal of Pharmacognosy.** V. 18, n.2, p. 314-319, 2008.

CASTILHO A.R., MURATA R.M.; PARDI, V. **Natural products in dentistry.** Health Magazine: 11-19, 2006.

CHARLES, D. J.; SIMON, J.E. A new geraniol chemotype of Ocimum gratissimum L. **Journal of essential oil research,** v. 4, p. 231-234, 1992.

CLINICAL AND LABORATORY STANDARDS INSTITUTE. Method for antifungal disk diffusion susceptibility testing of yeasts: approved Standard M44-A2. Wayne: **Clinical and Laboratory Standards Institute,** 2008a.

COLOMBO, A.L .; GUIMARÃES, T. Epidemiologia das infecções hematogénicas por *cândida* spp. **Revista da Sociedade Brasileira de Medicina Tropical,** Uberaba, v. 36, n.5, p. 599-607, sep-oct. 2003.

CORRÊA N. M, CARVALHO JÚNIOR F. B, IGNÁCIO R. F, LEONARDI G. R. Evaluation of the rheological behaviour of different hydrophilic gels. **Revista Brasileira de Ciências Farmacêuticas.** 2005; 41(1):73-8.

CHOW, J.K et al. Factors associated with candidemia caused by non-albicans Candida species versus *Candida albicans* in the intensive care unit. **Clinicai Infecious Diseases,** 46: 1206-1213, 2008.

DRAELOS, Z. D. **Cosmeceuticals.** Rio de Janeiro: Elsevier, 1991. 246 p.

DE PAULA, I.C.; ORTEGA, G.G.; BASSANI, V.L.; PETROVICK, P. R. Developmant of Ointment Formulations Prepared with Achyrocline satureioides Spray-Dried Extracts. **Drug Development and Industrial Pharmacy.** V.24, n.3, p.235-241, 1988.

DI STASI, L. C. et al. Medicinal plants popularly used in the Brazilian Tropical Atlantic Forest. **Fitoterapia,** v. 73, p. 69-91, 2002.

DUARTE, M. C. T. et al. Anti-Cand/da activity of Brazilian medicinal plants. **Journal of Ethnopharmacology,** v. 97, p. 305-311, 2005.

DUBEY, N.K. et al. Antifungal properties of Ocimum gratissimum essential oil (ethyl cinnamate chemotype). **Phytotherapy,** n.71, p.567-569, 2000

EHLERT, P. A. D.; LUZ, J. M. Q.; INNECCO, R. Vegetative propagation of carnation lavender using different types of cuttings and substrates. **Horticultura Brasileira,** v. 22, n.

1, p. 10-13, 2004.

FARMACOPÉIA BRASILEIRA, 4 ed. São Paulo: Atheneu, 2010.

FARIA, T. J. et al. *Ocimum gratissimum L.:* a rich source of ursolic acid and eugenol. In: Brazilian Conference on Natural Products, 1st, 2007, São Pedro. **Proceedings of the 1st BCNP.** São Pedro: Brazilian Chemical Society, 2007.

FERRARI, M. Development and evaluation of the photoprotective efficacy of multiple emulsions containing ethylhexyl methoxycinnamate and andiroba oil (Carapa guvanensis). 2002. 142p. **PhD Thesis in Pharmaceutical Sciences -** Ribeirão Preto School of Pharmaceutical Sciences, University of São Paulo, Ribeirão Preto.

FREIRE, C. M. M.; MARQUES, M. O. M.; COSTA, M.; **Journal of Ethnopharmacology.** 2006, 105, 161.

FLORENCE A. T.; ATTWOOD D. **Princípios Fisico-Químicos em Farmácia.** São Paulo: Editora da Universidade de São Paulo, p. 534-542, 2003.

FOLDVARI, M. Non-invasive administration of drugs through the skin: challenges in delivery system design. **Pharmaceutical Science & Technology Today,** v.3, n.12, p.417-425, 2000.

FRANCO, E. A. P.; BARROS, R. F. M. Use and diversity of medicinal plants in the Olho D'água dos Pires Quilombo, Esperantina, Piauí. **Revista Brasileira de Plantas Medicinais,** v. 8, n. 3, p. 78-88, 2006.

GALLEGOS, C., FRANCO, J.M. Rheology of food, cosmetics and pharmaceuticals. **Current Opinion in Colloid & Interface Science.** 1999; 4(4):288-93

GOODMAN, L. S.; GILMAN, A. **The Pharmacological Basis of Therapeutics.** Ed. Mc Graw Hill Interamericana do Brasil. ISBN 8577260011. Ed. 11a, 2006.

GARCIA, D., PUPO, S., CRESPO, M., FUENTES, L, 1998. Pharmacognostic study of *Ocimum gratissimum L.* (Orégano Cimarrón). Revista Cubana de Planta Medicinal, 31, 31-36.

GIOLO, M. P.; SVIDZINSKI T. I. E.; **Phisiopathogenesis, epidemiology and laboratory diagnosis of candidemia.** Brazilian Journal of Pathology and Laboratory Medicine, v. 46, n. 3, p. 225-234, 2010.

GOZALBO, D. et al. Candida and Candidiasis: The cell wall as a potential molecular target for antifungal therapy. **Current Drug Targets Infectious Disorders,** 4:117- 135, 2004.

GUENTHER, E. **The essential oils.** New York: D. Van Nostrand Company, 1948.

GUIRRO, E.; GUIRRO, R. **Dermo-Functional Physiopathology.** 3rd ed. São Paulo: Manole, 2002.

. **Dermato-functional physiotherapy.** 3. ed. Ver. Barueri: Manole, 2004.

HADCGRAFT J. Skin, the final frontier. **International Journal of Pharmaceutics,** Amsterdam, v.224,p.1-18, 2001.

HADCGRAFT J; LANE, E.M. Skin permeation: The years of enlightenment. **International Journal of Pharmaceutics,** v.305, p.2-12, 2005.

HAILLER, Virulence in Candida species. **Trends Microbiology,** 9: 591-596, 2011.

HAZEN, H.C.; New and emerging yeast pathogens. **Clinicai Microbiology.** 8:462- 478, 1995.

ISAAC, V. L. B.; CEFALI L. C.; CHIARI, B. G.; OLIVEIRA, C. C. L. G.; SALGADO H. R. N.; Corrêa, M. A. Protocol for physicochemical stability tests of phytocosmetics. **Revista de Ciências Farmacêuticas Básica e Aplicada,** v. 29, n. 1, p. 81-96, 2008.

IWU, M. M. **Handbook of African Medicinal Plants.** Florida: CRC Press Inc., 214215 p, 1993.

JIROVETZ, L. et al. Chemotaxonomic analysis of the essential oil aroma compounds of four different *Ocimum* species from Southern India. **European Food Research and Technology,** v. 217, p. 120-124, 2003.

JORGE M. H. A; EMERY, F. H; MORAES E SILVA, A. **Rooting of Lavender Cuttings** (Ocimum *gratissimum* L.). Corumbá: Embrapa Pantanal, 2006. 3 p. (Embrapa Pantanal. Technical Communication, 56).

JUNQUEIRA, L. C.; CARNEIRO, J. **Basic Histology.** 9th ed. São Paulo: Guanabara Koogan, 1999.

KOCSUBÉ S, TÓTH M, VÁGVOLGYI C, DÓCZI L, PESTI M, PÓCSI I et al. Occurrence and genetic variability of *Candida parapsilosis* sensu lato in Hungary. **Journal of Medical Microbiology** 2007; 56: 190-195.

KOMMANABOYINA, B.; RHODES, C.T. Trends in stability testing, with emphasis on stability during distribution and storage. **Drug Development and Industrial Pharmacy,** v. 25, p. 857-868, 1999.

KOROLKOVAS, A. **Guanabara Therapeutic Dictionary.** Ed. 2001/2002, Guanabara Koogan, Rio de Janeiro.

KORTING, S. M.; MEHNERT, W.; KORTING, H. C.; Lipid nanoparticles for improved topical application of drugs for skin diseases. **Advanced Drug Delivery Reviews,** v. 59, p. 427- 443, 2007.

KRETSOS, K. *et.al.* Partitioning, diffusivity and clearance of skin permeants in mammalian dermis. **International Journal of Pharmaceutics,** v.346, p. 64-79, 2008.

LABA, D. **Rheological properties of cosmetics and toiletries.** New York: Mareei Dekker; 1993. p.9-33.

LAFFEY SF, BUTLER G. Phenotype swiching affects bioflm formatio by *Candida parapsilosis.* **Microbiology** 2005; 151: 1073-1081

LEMOS, J. et al. Antifungal activity from *Ocimum gratissimum L.* towards *Cryptococcus neoformans.* **Memórias do Instituto Oswaldo Cruz,** Rio de Janeiro, v.100, p. 55-58, 2005.

LEONARDI, G.R, MAIA CAMPOS PMBG. Stability of cosmetic formulations. **International Journal of Pharmaceutical Compounding.** Ed Bras. 2001; 3(4):154- 6.

LEONARDI, G. R.; MARTINS, L. G.; KUREBAYASHI, M. **Skin permeation. Cosmetologia aplicada,** São Paulo: Medfarma, 2004.

Leonardi, Gislaine R.; Campos, Patrícia M.B.G.M. Hidratação cutânea. **Revista Brasileira de Farmácia.** n° 30 (1/2/3). p. 77-78, 2002.

LI L, REDDING S, DONGARI-BAGTZOGLOU A. *Candida glabrata,* an emergingoral opportunistic pathogen. **Journal of Dental Research** 2007; 86(3): 204-215.

LIMA, C. B.; BELLETTINI, N. M. T.; SILVA, A. S.; CHEIRUBIM, A. P.; JANANI, J. K.; VIEIRA, M. A. V.; AMADOR, T. S. Uso de Plantas Medicinais pela população da zona urbana de Bandeirantes- PR. **Brazilian Journal of Biosciences,** v. 5, p. 600602, 2007.

LIMA, I. O.; OLIVEIRA, R. A. G.; LIMA, E. O.; FARIAS, N. M. P.; SOUZA, E. L. Antifungal activity of essential oils on Candida species. **Brazilian Journal of Pharmacognosy,** 2006.

LIMA, C. G., VILELA, A. F. G, SILVA, A. A. S., PIANNOVSKI, A. R., SILVA, K. K., CARVALHO, V. F. M" MUSIS, C. R" MACHADO, S. R. P" FERRARI, M. Development and evaluation of the physical stability of O/W emulsions containing babassu oil (Orb/gnya *oleifera).* **Revista Brasileira de Farmacognosia,** 89 (3): 239245, 2008.

LUPETTI A, TAVANTI A, DAVINI P, GHELARDI E, CORSINI V, MERUSI I et al. Horizontal transmission of Candida parapsilosis candidemia in a neonatal intensive care unit. **Journal of Clinical Microbiology** 2002; 40(7): 2363-2369.

LORENZI H.; MATOS F. J. A. **Plantas Medicinais do Brasil: nativas e exóticas.** São Paulo: Instituto Plantarum de Estudos da Flora, 512p, 2000.

MANOSROI, A., JANTRAWUT, P., MANOSRI, J. Anti-inflammatory activity of gel containing novel elastic niosomes with diclofenac diethylammonium. **International Journal of Pharmaceutics.** v. 360, p.156-163, 2008.

MARTINS, R. M, CORTEZ, L. E. R., FELIPE, D. F. Development of topical formulations using essential oil extracted from cloves. **Revista de Saúde e Pesquisa,** v. 1, n. 3, p. 259-263, Sep./Dec. 2008.

MARTINS, A. P" SALGUEIRO, L.R., VILA, R" TOMI, F" CANIGUERAL, S" CASANOVA, J., CUNHA, A.P., ADZET, T., 1999. Composition of the essential oils of Ocimum canun, O. gratissimum and O. minimum. **Planta Medica.** 65, 187-189.

MATASYOH L. G.; MATASYOH J. C.; WACHIRA F. N.; KINYUA M. G.; THAIRU A. W. M.; MUKIAMA T. K. Chemical composition and antimicrobial activity of tho essential oil of *Ocimum gratissimum* L. growing in Eastern Kenya. **African Journal of Biotechnology,** 6: 760-765, 2007.

MATOS, F. J. A. **Farmácias vivas.** Fortaleza: Editora da Universidade Federal do Ceará, 55-56 p, 1994.

MATOS, F. J.A. **Farmácias Vivas: a** system for the utilisation of medicinal plants designed for small communities. 3. ed. Fortaleza: EUFC, 1998. 220p.

MIGUEL, M. D.; MIGUEL, O. G.. **Development of herbal medicines.** São Paulo: Robe, 1999.

MILLER, D., WIENER, E.M, TUROWSKI, A., THUNING, C" HOFFMANN, H., O/W emulsions for cosmetics products stabilised by alkyl phosphates - rheology and storage tests. **Colloids Surf A Physicochemical and Engineering Aspects.** 1999; 152(1-2): 155-60

MIYAZAKI, S.; A. TAKAHASHI, W. KUBO, J. BACHYNSKY & R. LÖBENBERG. **Journal of Pharmaceutical Sciences,** v. 6, p. 238-245, 2003.

MONTALVO, R. V.; DOMÍNGUEZ, C. C. Efecto sobre la motilidad intestinal y toxicidad aguda del extracto fluido de *Ocimum gratissimum* L. (Orégano cimarrón). **Revista Cubana de Plantas Medieinales,** v. 2, n. 2-3, p. 14-18, 1997.

MORAIS, S. M.; DANTAS, J. D. P.; SILVA, A. R. A; MAGALHAES, E. F. Medicinal plants used by the Tapebas Indians of Ceará. **Revista Brasileira de Farmacognosia,** 15: 169-177, 2005.

MOORE, K. L.; DARLLY, A. F. **Clinically orientated anatomy.** 4. ed. Rio de Janeiro: Guanabara, 2001.

MORGANTI, P.; RUOCCO, E.; WOLF, R.; RUOCCO, V. Percutaneous absorption in delivery systems. **Clinicai Dermatology,** v. 19, p. 489-501, 2001.

MOSTEFA, N. M; SADOK, A. H.; SABRI, N.; HADJI, A. Determination of optimal cream formulation from long-term stability investigation using a surface response modelling. **International Journal of Cosmetic Science,** v. 28, n. 3, p. 211-218, 2006.

MCMANUS BA, COLEMAN DC, MORAN G, PINJON E, DIOGO D, BOUGNOUX ME et al. Multilocus sequence typing reveals that the population structure of *Candida dubliniensis* is significantly less divergent than that of *Candida albicans.* **Journal Clinicai Microbiology** 2008; 46(2): 652-664.

NAGLIK, J. et al. ***Candida albicans* proteinases and host/pathogen interactions.** Cell. Microbiol., 6(10):915-926, 2004.

NAKAMURA, C. V. et al. Antibacterial Activity of *Ocimum gratissimum L.* Essential Oil. **Memórias do Instituto Oswaldo Cruz,** Rio de Janeiro, v. 94, n. 5, p. 674-678, 1999.

NIERO, R.; MALHEIROS, A.; BITTENCOURT, C. M. S.; BIAVATTI, M. W.; LEITE, S. N. Chemical and biological aspects of medicinal plants and considerations on phytotherapics. In: BRESOLIN, T. M. B.; CHECHINEL FILHO, V. (Org.). **Pharmaceutical Sciences:** contribution to the development of new drugs and medicines. Itajaí: Univali, p. 10-56, 2003.

NJOKU, C. J. et al. Oleanolic acid, a bioactive component of the leaves of *Ocimum gratissimum* (Lamiaceae). **International Journal of Pharmacognosy, v.** 35, n. 2, p. 134-137, 1997.

OFFIAH, V.N., CHIKWENDU, U.A.,1999. Antidiarrhoeal effects of Ocimum gratissimum leaf extract in experimental animals. **Journal of Ethnopharmacology.** 68, 327-330.

OUX SS, CATIA G, MARZIA I, FRANCESCO VF, AFOUXBI AA, NADIA M. HPLC/DAD/MS characterisation and analysis of flavonoids and cynnamoil derivatives in four Nigerian green-leafy vegetables. **Food Chemistry** v.115, p 1568-1574, 2009.

OLIVEIRA, A. C. Herbal **medicine:** phytochemical profile, control and validation of analytical methodology. 2005. Master's dissertation. Federal University of Pernambuco, Recife, 2005.

OLIVEIRA, C. J.; ARAÚJO, T. L. Medicinal plants: uses and beliefs of enderly carriers of arterial hypertension. **Revista Eletrónica de Enfermagem,** v. 9, p. 93105, 2007.

OLIVEIRA, D. A. G. C.; DUTRA, E. A.; SANTORO, M. I. R. M.; HACKMANN, E. R. M. K. Sunscreens, Radiation and Skin. **Cosmetics & Toiletries** (Portuguese Edition), v.16, p.68-72, Mar/April, 2004.

OLIVEIRA, V. B. et al. Native foods from Brazilian biodiversity as source of bioactive compounds. **Food Research International,** v. 48, p. 170-179, 2012.

ONAJOBI, F. D. Smooth muscle contracting lipid-soluble principies in chromatographic fractions of *Ocimum gratissimum.* **Journal of Ethnopharmacology,** v. 18, p. 03-11, 1986.

PALMA, M.; GIUDICI, R. Emulsion copolymerisation of vinyl acetate and butyl acrylate with high solids content. **Polymers: Science and Technology; v.** 16; n° 004; p. 269-275; 2006.

PALMEIRA FILHO, P. L.; PAN, S. S. K. Cadeia farmacêutica no Brasil: avaliação preliminar e perspectivas. **BNDES Setorial,** Rio de Janeiro, n. 18, p. 3-22, Sep. 2003.

PATON, A. J. et al. Phylogeny and evolution of basils and allies (Ocimeae, Labiatae) based on three plastid DNA regions. **Molecular Phylogenetics and Evolution,** v. 31, p. 277-299, 2004.

PENA, L.E, LEE, B.L, STEATNS, J.F. Consistency development and destabilisation of a model cream. **Journal of the Society of Cosmetic Chemists.** 1993; 44(6):337- 45.

PEREIRA, D. C., FRASSON, A. P. Z. Use of *Aloe Vera* in pharmaceutical products and analysis of the physicochemical stability of anionic cream containing glycolic extract of this plant. **Revista Contexto & Saúde,** v. 6, n. 12, Ijuí-RS, 2007.

PENTEADO FILHO, S. R. Antimicrobial control: theory, evidence and practice. **Hospital Practice,** v. 36, p. 8-12, 2004.

PEREIRA, C. A. M; MAIA, J. F. Estudo da atividade antioxidante do extrato e do óleo essencial obtido das folhas de alfavaca (Ocimum gratissimum L.). **Ciência e Tecnologia de Alimentos,** campinas, v. 27, n. 3, p.91-97, 2007. 2007.

PIANOVSKI, A. R., VILELA, A. F. G., SILVA, A. A. S., LIMA, C. G., SILVA, K. K., CARVALHO, V. F. M" MUSIS, C. R" MACHADO, S. R. P" FERRARI, M. Use of pequi oil *(Caryocar brasiliense)* in cosmetic emulsions: development and evaluation of physical stability. **Revista Brasileira de Ciências Farmacêuticas,** v. 44, n. 2, Cuiabá-MT, 2008.

PFALLER, M. A. et al. *Candida glabrata:* **Multidrug Resistance and Increased Virulence in a Major Opportunistic Fungai Pathogen.** Current Fungai Infection Reports, 6: 154-164, 2012.

PFALLER MA, DIEKEMA DJ, GIBBS DL, NEWELL VA, NAGY E, DOBIASOVAS et al.

Candida krusei, a multidrug-resistant opportunistic fungal pathogen: geographic and temporal trends from the ARTEMIS DISK antifungal surveillance programme, 2001 to 2005. **Journal of Medical Microbiology** 2008; 46(2): 515-521.

PROENÇA, K.S.; ROMA, R.M.; OLIVEIRA, R.V.M.; GONÇALVES, M.; VILA, M.M.D.C. Evaluation of the stability of creams using different consistency agents. **Revista Brasileira de Farmácia,** 87th ed; n.3; p. 74-77, 2006.

RABELO, M. et al. Antinociceptive properties of the essential oil of *Ocimum gratissimum L.* (Labiatae) in mice. **Brazilian Journal of Medicine and Biological Research,** v. 36, p. 521-524, 2003.

Rieger, Martin M. Emulsions. In: Lachman, L.; Lieberman, H.A.; Kanig, J.L. **Teoria e prática na Indústria Farmacêutica,** v. II. Lisboa: Calouste Gulbenkian, 2001. p. 856. 894 - 902

SAAVEDRA, M. J. Antibiotic resistance of the genus *Aeromonas* spp. **Aquaculture Research & Development,** v.3, n. 2, doi: 10.4172/2155-9546.1000e101, 2012.

SAINSBURY, M" SOFOWORA, E.A., 1971. Essential oil from the leaves and inflorescence of Ocimum gratissimum. Phytochemistry 10, 3309-3310.

SOMASUNDARAN, P" MEHTA, S. C" PUROHIT, P. Silicone emulsions. **Advances in Colloid and Interface Science,** v. 21, n. 128-139, p. 103-109, 2007.

SARTORATTO, A. et al. Composition and antimicrobial activity of essential oils from aromatic plants used in Brazil. **Brazilian Journal of Microbiology,** v. 35, p. 275-280, 2004.

SILVA, L. L.; HELDWEIN, C. G" REETZ, L. G. B.; HORNER, R.; MALLMANN, C. A.; HEINZMANN, B. M. Chemical composition, *in vitro* antibacterial activity and toxicity in *Artemia salina of* the essential oil from the inflorescences of *Ocimum gratissimum* L., Lamiaceae. **Revista Brasileira de Farmacognosia,** 20(5): 700-705, Oct./Nov, 2010.

SILVA, M. I. G.; GONDIM, A. P. S.; NUNES, I. F.; SOUSA, F. C. F. Utilisation of herbal medicines in basic family health care units in the municipality of Maracanaú (CE). **Revista Brasileira de Farmacognosia,** 16: 455-462, 2006.

SILVA, V. A.; FREITAS, A. F. R.; PEREIRA, M. S. V.; OLIVEIR, C.R. M.; DINIZ, M. F. F. M.; PESSÔA, H. L. F. Antifungal efficacy of extracts of *Lippia sidoides Cham.* and *Matricaria recutita Linn.* on yeasts of the *Candida* genus. **Journal of Biology and Pharmacy,** Vol. 05, No. 1, 2011.

SILVA, M. A . S; PEREIRA, M. S; ANDRADE. E; CIGOLINI, C. A; MARQUES, **M.O.M. Efeito da época de colheita sobre a produção de biomassa, rendimento e composição do óleo essencial de *Ocimum gratissimum L. sob as* condições do norte do Mato Grosso.** In: Brazilian Symposium on Essential Oils, 4, 2007, Fortaleza. Abstracts. Fortaleza: Agronomic Institute of Campinas, 2007.

SILVA, S. M. F. Q. et al. In vitro activity of crude extracts of two plant species from the cerrado on yeasts of the genus Candida. **Ciências da saúde coletiva [Online],** 17(6): 1649-1656, 2012

SILVEIRA, L. M. S.; OLEA, R. S. G.; MESQUITA, J. S.; CRUZ, A. DE L. N.; MENDES,J. C. Antimicrobial activity methodology applied to plant extracts: comparison between two agar diffusion techniques. **Revista Brasileira de Farmacologia,** 90 (2): 124-128, 2009.

SIMÕES, C. M. O.; SCHENKEL, E. P.; GOSMANN, G.; MELLO, J. C. P.; MENTZ, L. A.; PETROVICK, P. R. **Farmacognosia:** da planta ao medicamento. 5. ed. Porto Alegre: UFRGS, 2003.

SINKO, J.P., **Martin: physical pharmacy and pharmaceutical sciences.** São Paulo: Editora Artmed, 809 p, 2008.

SCHOTT, H. Rheology. In: Gennaro AR (ed) Remington: the Science and practice of Pharmacia. 19th ed. Pennsylvania: **Mack Publishing Company;** 1995. p.426-55.

TADROS, T. Application of rheology for assessment and prediction of the long-tem physical stability of emulsions. **Ady Colloid Interface Sei** 2004; 108:227-58.

TAMBURIC S. The aging of polymer-stabilised creams: **A rheological viewpoint. Cosmet Toilet.** 2000; 115(10):43-9.

TOLEDO, A. C.; HIRATA, L.L.; BUFFON, M. C. M.; MIGUEL, M. D.; MIGUEL, O. G. Phytotherapics: a pharmacotechnical approach. **Revista Lecta,** v. 21, n. 1/2, p.7-13, 2003.

TCHOUMBOUGNANG, F" AMVAM ZOLLO, P.H., AVIESSI, F" ALITONOU, G.A., SOHOUNHLOUE, D.K., OUAMBA, J.M., TROMAMBET, A., ANDISSA, N.O., DAGNE, E" AGNANIET, H" BESSIÈRE, J.M., MENUT, C" 2006. Variability in the Chemical compositions of the essential oils of five *Ocimum* Species from Tropical African Area. **Journal of Essential Oil Research.** 18, 194-199

UEDA-NAKAMURA, T. et al. Antileishmanial activity of Eugenol-rich essential oil from *Ocimum gratissimum.* **Parasitology International,** v.55, n.2, p.99-105, 2006.

VERMA, D. D.; VERMA, S.; BLUME, G.; FAHR, A. Particle size of liposomes influences dermal delivery of substances into skin. **International Journal of Pharmaceutics,** v. 258, (1-2), p. 141-151, 2003.

VIEIRA, R. et al. Use of chemical markers in the study of the genetic diversity of Ocimum gratissimum L. **Revista Brasileira de Farmacognosia,** v. 12, p. 126-129, 2002.

VIEIRA, R.F., GRAYER, R.J., PATON, A., SIMON, J.E., 2001. Genetic diversity of *Ocimum gratissimum L.* based on volatile oil constituents, flavonoids and RAPD markers. **Biochemical Systematics and Ecology.** 29, 287-304.

YAYI, E" GBENOU, J.D., AHOUSSI, L.A., MOUDACHIROU, M" CHALCHAT, J.C., 2004. Ocimum gratissimum L., siège de variations chimiques complexes au cours du développement. **Comptes Rendus Chimie** 7, 1013-1018

ZIMERMAN, R. A. **Indiscriminate Use of Antimicrobials and Microbial Resistance.** In: Brazil. Ministry of Health. Secretariat for Science, Technology and Strategic Inputs. Rational use of medicines: selected themes / Ministry of Health, Secretariat of Science, Technology and Strategic Inputs - Brasília: Ministry of Health, 2012.

WOLFFENBÚTTEL, A. N. **Essential Oils,** 2007. Available at: <http://www.oleoessencial.com.br/artigo_Adriana.pdf>. Accessed on: 19 September 2014.

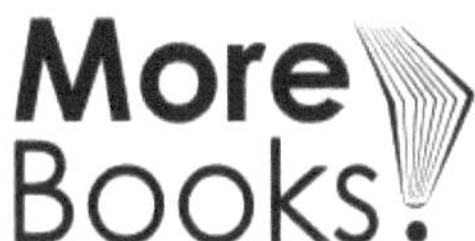

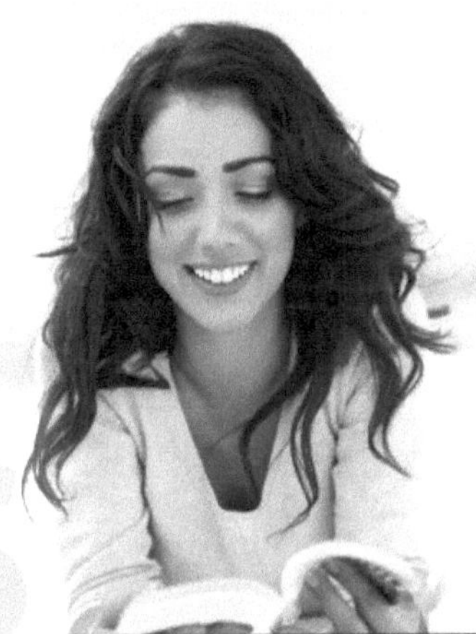

I want morebooks!

Buy your books fast and straightforward online - at one of world's fastest growing online book stores! Environmentally sound due to Print-on-Demand technologies.

Buy your books online at
www.morebooks.shop

Kaufen Sie Ihre Bücher schnell und unkompliziert online – auf einer der am schnellsten wachsenden Buchhandelsplattformen weltweit! Dank Print-On-Demand umwelt- und ressourcenschonend produziert.

Bücher schneller online kaufen
www.morebooks.shop

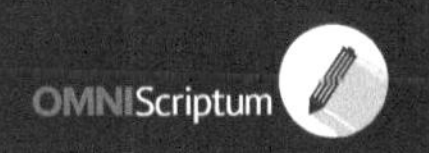